DON'T

In Control of
Fear, Panic & Anxiety

EVE RUSSELL

Author of the best selling tape

First published in Great Britain 2001

Published by Feelgood Publications

PO Box 2, Stockport, SK4 3FU United Kingdom

Copyright ©2001 Feelgood

The moral right of the author has been asserted

All rights reserved

No part of this publication may be reproduced, stored in a retrieval system, or transmitted, in any form or by any means without the prior written permission of the publisher, nor be otherwise circulated in any form of binding or cover other than that in which it is published and without a similar condition including this condition being imposed on the subsequent purchaser

The author and publisher advise the reader to check with a doctor before undertaking any course of treatment or exercise and take no responsibility for any possible consequences arising from following the information in this book.

ISBN: 0-9541871-0-5

Graphic Design Garry Behling

Printed in England by William Clowes Ltd.

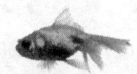

ACKNOWLEDGMENTS

To my husband & daughter. Thank you for your endless understanding love support and inspiration.

To our families. Thank you all for your encouragement love and support.

To my Junior School Teacher, David Cox who taught us how to create magic with thoughts and words and who saw the potential in all of us not just the few.

To Garry for always being ready to help unconditionally. Thanks Gaz

To Marlene. Thank you

To all my friends - you know who you are

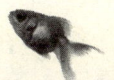

INTRODUCTION

In 1995 I produced an audio tape 'In Control of Panic & Anxiety'. The letters I received as a result of this tape confirmed how many people live in a state of constant fear, panic and anxiety. As someone who has personal experience of panic attacks I know only too well how the frightening and overwhelming symptoms of dizziness, feelings of unreality, shallow breathing, a sense that something awful is going to happen, can affect our family social and work life.

The feelings often appear out of the blue and because of this we begin to avoid doing things which once gave us pleasure, a trip to the cinema, a meal out, going to the airport to begin our holidays, or going shopping. Fear can be so disabling that for some people it becomes virtually impossible to leave the house.

Many people feel isolated and unable to talk about how they feel because of a fear that others will see them as weak or simply imagining the symptoms. I would like to reassure you that although you may feel isolated you are definitely not alone and the feelings you are having are real and deserve to be recognised.

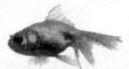

We live in stressful and anxious times. As well as the things that are going on in our own personal lives we are also affected by the things going on in the world around us.

Sometimes it seems that whichever way we turn there is a reason to be frightened.

My hope by writing this little book is that you will find something in it which will offer you some practical help, comfort and calm.

I don't claim to know all the answers but I do know that if we can begin to understand why these feelings overtake us, treat ourselves gently, have patience and start trying to untie the knots inside us, we can hope to see changes in the way we feel.

This book is not intended as a substitute for any medical treatment or counselling you may be having, but comes to you as a friend who knows how you are feeling and wants to offer some support.

With love and best wishes

Eve Russell

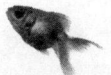

FEAR

fear is a basic and perfectly natural human response to something we find threatening. It has been part of us since time began and helps us to protect ourselves from dangerous situations.

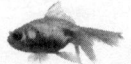

FIGHT OR FLIGHT

when we need to run away from danger our body takes on the 'fight or flight' response and a flood of adrenaline is released into the body preparing us for action - helping us to deal with the threat.

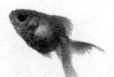

NO DANGER

feelings of fear and panic can also take over when there is no obvious danger to us as individuals. This can often lead to a state of constant apprehension which can affect our quality of life.

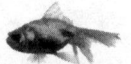

TRAPPED BY FEAR

it's easy to get caught up in a trap of fear. The uncertainty of what might happen to us feeds our anxieties.

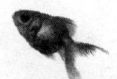

RELEASING STRESS

panic and anxiety symptoms are usually the result of an over production of adrenaline in the bloodstream and are the body's way of releasing stress which may have gone unrecognised for a long time.

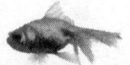

OUT OF THE BLUE

these feelings can come out of the blue or you may have had them for some time.

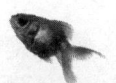

OVERWHELMING SYMPTOMS

the symptoms are often very frightening and can be so overwhelming that it's easy to feel that something terrible is going to happen. The fear of losing control particularly in public places begins to overtake us.

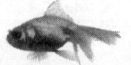

SEEMS LIKE FOREVER

although it seems to be forever, remember that most panic attacks will only last for between 5 and 20 minutes.

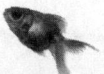

RECOGNISE YOUR FEELINGS

whether or not you know the reasons for your fear, panic and anxiety, it is important to recognise that the feelings you are having are REAL.

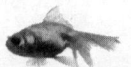

YOU ARE NOT WEAK

being scared doesn't EVER mean that you are weak. It simply means that you are human.

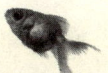

YOU ARE NOT ALONE

you may be feeling isolated but you are certainly not alone. Everyone experiences fear and nearly 1 in 5 people of all ages and from all walks of life experience panic and anxiety symptoms.

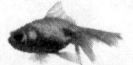

TENSING UP

when we are scared our first reaction is to tense up and tighten a body which is already anxious.

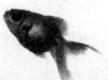

OVERBREATHING

feelings of fear often cause us to overbreathe resulting in a drop in the levels of carbon dioxide in the body.

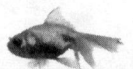

UNTIE THE KNOTS

this can make the symptoms of fear and panic feel even worse and begin to create a vicious circle. This can be hard to come out of unless we learn how to untie the knots.

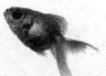

SLOW DOWN

try and slow down your breathing.

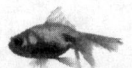

UNDERSTANDING

understanding and accepting the cause and nature of your anxiety is often the beginning of recovery.

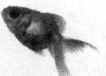

PUBLIC PLACES

for many of us the greatest fear of all is of losing control in a public place, of passing out and making a fool of ourselves in front of others. Remember the mechanisms which cause us to faint are quite different to those which cause us to panic.

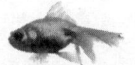

DON'T BE ASHAMED

it's easy to create your own stigma about your feelings of fear, panic and anxiety. Remember you are not weak because you get them. They are nothing to be ashamed of.

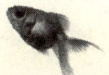

GET YOUR FEELINGS OUT

it is helpful to get your feelings out into the open and talk about them to someone you trust and who you know will support and listen to you.

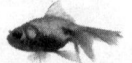

BOTTLING UP OUR FEELINGS

when we bottle up our feelings we deprive ourselves of the support we could otherwise have.

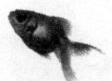

ACCEPT YOUR FEELINGS

although it's not always easy to do, try and accept your physical and emotional feelings as the symptoms of being scared.

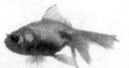

FEAR IS JUST A FEELING

hard as it may be to believe, fear is just a feeling.

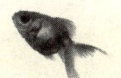

LOOK AT FEAR
FACE TO FACE

fear often loses its power if you can look at it face to face, accept it, name it and share your concerns with someone else.

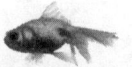

FEAR OF PUBLIC PLACES

supermarkets, shops, meetings, cinemas, restaurants and other busy places are often where the panic and fear feelings overtake us and our immediate reaction is to run away.

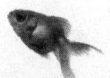

STOP!

when the lights are too bright, when the noise is too loud when the fear is too much. STOP!

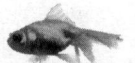

DROP YOUR SHOULDERS

drop your shoulders breathe in as deeply as you can, hold the breath for a few seconds and then slowly release it.

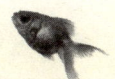

BREATHE

or cup your hands over your mouth and nose and breathe normally for a few minutes.

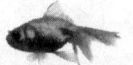

SIT QUIETLY

if there is a window in the building where natural daylight comes in, just quietly go and stand or sit by it for a while.

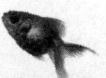

YOU HAVE NOT FAILED

if the need to go outside is overwhelming there is nothing wrong with this. It doesn't mean that you've failed.

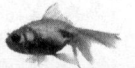

PANIC WILL SUBSIDE

take your time.
Remember the body is self regulating.

Fear and panic will always subside
if we allow it to.

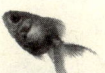

ENCOURAGE YOURSELF

try and gently encourage yourself to go back into the situation. With practice this can be really helpful in reducing the feelings of fear.

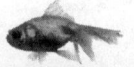

TELL SOMEONE

remember it is perfectly alright for you to tell the person you are with, or someone else, that you get panicky feelings.

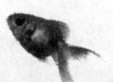

OFFERING SUPPORT

most people will want to offer support and you'll be surprised at how many will identify with your symptoms or know someone that gets them.

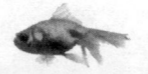

I AM SAFE

positive self talk such as 'I am alright', 'I am safe' can be really helpful if repeated on a regular basis and especially when the panic feelings begin.

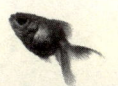

FEELINGS OF ANGER

you may be feeling angry or frustrated at how the feelings of fear, panic and anxiety are affecting your life.

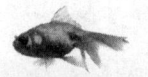

ANGER IS PERFECTLY NATURAL

anger is a perfectly natural response to something we feel we don't have any control over.

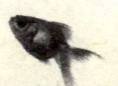

WRITE YOUR ANGER DOWN

tell someone you trust that you feel angry or write your feelings down on paper.

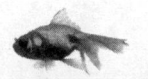

MAKING POSITIVE CHANGES

anger can sometimes give us the chance to get a clearer picture of what is important to us and can help us to make positive changes in our lives.

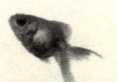

HAVE A MASSAGE

have a shoulder or neck massage on a regular basis, tension often makes its home here. Ask someone you love and trust to do this for you.

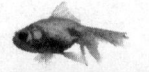

YOUR BODY IS YOUR FRIEND

try and think of your body as your friend not your enemy.

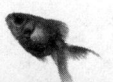

COVERING UP

covering up the symptoms of fear makes the anxiety worse and creates more tension in our bodies.

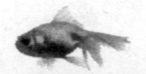

RELAX YOUR BODY

the more relaxed your body is the harder it is for the panic to take over.

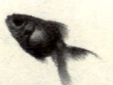

TEARS ARE CLEANSING

when you feel angry, frustrated, sad or just simply fed up, allow yourself to cry, tears are cleansing and release pent up anxieties and emotions.

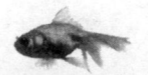

A MOMENT IN TIME

today is a moment in time, accept the way you feel right now, go with the flow stay with the fear. Don't start a war with your body.

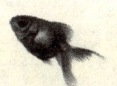

JUST FOR TODAY

just for today don't worry, just for today don't anger, just for today don't judge.

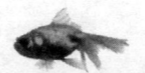

HELP

*you don't have to suffer in silence.
there are organisations and groups
who can give you support and who
want to help.*

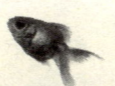

PROTECTING PEOPLE WE LOVE

it's a natural human response to want to protect the people we care about from our worries and this can sometimes lead to a breakdown in communication and deprive us of the support we could otherwise have.

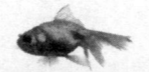

ASK FOR HELP

ask for help from your partner, your doctor, your friends, God or the Universe, whoever you believe in and trust.

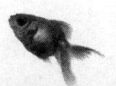

STRENGTH

remember asking for help is a sign of STRENGTH not of weakness.

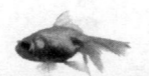

PLEASING OTHERS

learn how to say no. Many of us put ourselves under added stress by trying to please others and neglect our own needs in the process.

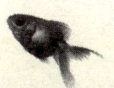

PEOPLE WHO CARE WILL UNDERSTAND

the people who really care about you and want to help you will understand if you say no to certain things.

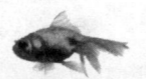

YOU ARE NOT SELFISH

allow yourself time to do things that give YOU pleasure. This doesn't mean that you are being selfish.

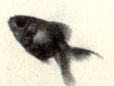

RECOGNISE YOUR OWN NEEDS

it simply means that you are recognising your own needs and doing something positive to help yourself.

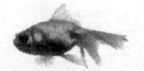

KEEPING COMPANY WITH PEOPLE YOU LIKE

as far as possible keep the company of people who you like being with and who make you feel good about yourself. Many of us spend too much time and energy worrying about what others think of us.

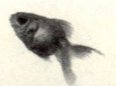

WE ARE ALL INDIVIDUALS

remember we are all individuals with different ways of dealing with things.

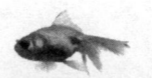

YOU DON'T HAVE TO BE A HERO

you don't have to be a hero, you don't have to be perfect. Just do what you can for now.

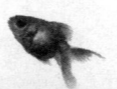

SWITCH OFF FROM THE NEGATIVE

in these changing times it is easy to absorb all the negative news around us. Learn to switch off from the negative and try to concentrate on the pleasant and good things going on around you.

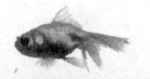

A FLOWER BLOOMING

*a flower blooming, a baby's smile,
a bird singing, a hug from someone
you love.*

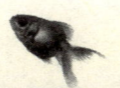

SMILING

smile as much as you can. Smiling helps to get rid of tension and gives us a good feeling inside.

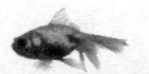

WATCH A FUNNY FILM

listen to your favourite music, dance, play a game, watch a funny film, watch a sad film.

Take a chair outside and sit in the fresh air.

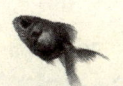

THE PRESENT

the past may be full of knocks, bruises and heartache. It is all water under the bridge. Look to the present and the future.

Nature moves only forward.

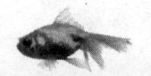

CREATE A PICTURE

create a picture in your mind, see yourself as you would like to be, **HAPPY, CALM, RELAXED FREE FROM FEAR, PANIC & ANXIETY** *Keep this picture with you. Look at it regularly.*

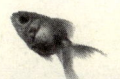

EATING AND DRINKING

keep a record of what you eat and drink. Too much sugar, caffeine and alcohol can bring on or increase our feelings of panic.

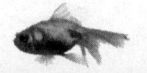

FOOD

eating healthy food at regular intervals is important for blood sugar levels. A vitamin B complex supplement can often help a stressed out nervous system as can drinking lots of water.

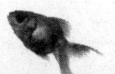

RESCUE REMEDY

many people find Dr Bachs Rescue Remedy helpful. Put a few drops on your tongue when you feel the fear taking over.

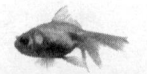

DESIDERATA

*'Many fears are born of imaginings'
(Desiderata). Many of our worries are
about things that will never happen.*

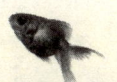

WALK AROUND YOUR GARDEN

even if you are not able to venture far from your home for now, regular exercise is really helpful. Walk around your garden, round the block or to the end of the road and back.

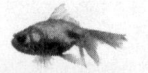

HUM TO YOURSELF

if you are out and feel fear or panic coming over you try and take a deep a breath into your stomach and make a humming sound as you breathe out. This is particularly good if you are walking.

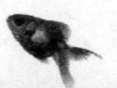

OILS AND TEA

to ease anxiety, the essential oils Bergamot, Lavender, Jasmine Ylang Ylang and Rosewood are all helpful. Lemon balm tea is particularly good at providing comfort and uplifting the spirits. It can also help to reduce feelings of nervousness, panic and quieten a racing heart.

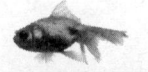

VISUALISE YELLOW

visualise and breathe in the colour yellow. This calming colour helps to reduce feelings of panic.

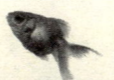

BE KIND TO YOURSELF

set aside 10 minutes in the morning and evening to be quiet, kind and loving to yourself. Unplug the phone, switch off the TV. Just sit as calmly as you can and simply observe your breathing.

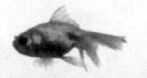

BREATHE IN HAPPINESS

*as you breathe in, take in happiness,
peace and light. As you breathe out,
release all the anxiety, tension and fear.
Visualise yourself as you would like
to be.*

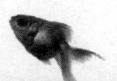

UNTIE THE KNOTS

in bed at night lie in a comfortable position. Breathe in and tense all the muscles in your body one by one, hold the tension for a few seconds and then breathe out. Try and do this on a regular basis.

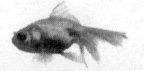

THE JOURNEY SEEMS LONG

there may be days when everything seems impossible. The journey seems long, the roads are complicated and sometimes there are just too many traffic lights.

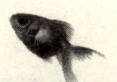

YOU ARE IN CONTROL

have patience, have perseverance, have trust, take comfort, be calm.

YOU are in control.

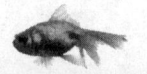

FOR FAMILY AND FRIENDS

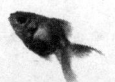

FRUSTRATION

you may be feeling frustrated and resentful at how the fear has affected not only the life of someone you care about but also your own.

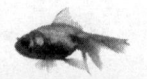

FEELINGS ARE NATURAL

please recognise that these feelings are perfectly natural.

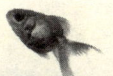

ENCOURAGE DISCUSSION

try to encourage your family member or friend to describe how they feel. This will help you to understand that the feelings are very real.

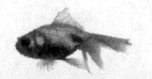

HOW CAN I HELP

ask how you can help and give support.

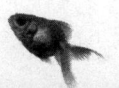

TALKING

allowing yourself to talk about how you feel is equally as important and often helps to clear the air.

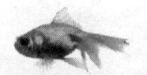

EMOTIONAL TIMETABLE

however we don't always operate on the same emotional timetable. Sometimes a hug, a smile or just holding hands are ways in which we can receive or offer support without saying a word.

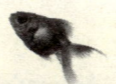

CALM MANNER

a calm relaxed and reassuring manner is really helpful.

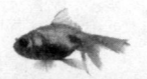

OFFERING COMPROMISES

offer compromises in social situations where you know the feelings of fear and panic are particularly bad for the person you care about, but also try to gently encourage them to stay in these situations for as long as possible.

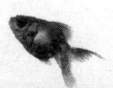

HELPFUL STATEMENTS

statements like 'everything's alright' and 'you're safe' can really help to reduce feelings of fear and panic.

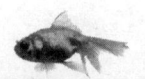

GOALS

work together on goals and targets to encourage small steps forward.

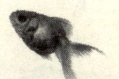

LAUGH

try and introduce some humour into the situation so that things don't always have to feel so serious.

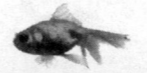

PLEASURE

don't lose sight of your own needs and aim to do things which you enjoy and give you pleasure and relaxation.

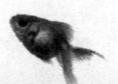

YOU ARE NOT BEING SELFISH

this doesn't mean that you are being selfish.

Remember you will be able to offer support more easily if your own needs are not being neglected.

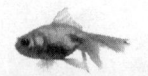

LIGHTEN THE LOAD

*have patience, trust and perseverance,
The load may seem heavy but sharing it
makes it a lot lighter.
Your encouragement and support is
greatly valued and appreciated.*

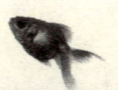

HELPFUL ORGANISATIONS

NATIONAL PHOBICS SOCIETY
ZION COMMUNITY RESOURCE CENTRE
339 STRETFORD RD HULME
MANCHESTER M15 42Y
TEL: 0870 7700456

NO PANIC
93 BRANDS FARM WAY
TELFORD SHROPSHIRE TF3 2JQ
HELPLINE NUMBER: 01952 590545

A FEELGOOD PUBLICATION COPYRIGHT ©2001

FOR FURTHER INFORMATION ABOUT FEELGOOD PUBLICATIONS PLEASE CONTACT

P.O BOX 2 STOCKPORT SK4 3FU U.K.

The audio tape 'In Control of Panic & Anxiety' is available in the U.K. from the above address for £7.99 (inc p&p).

Further copies of this book are available for £2.99 (inc p&p). Cheques or postal orders should be made payable to Feelgood.

All information correct at the time of publishing.

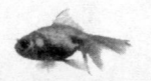